P

Andrew exudes a quiet confidence, warmth and expertise to both audiences and clients when he discusses the impact of untreated hearing loss on brain health; he is at the forefront of all the latest research on the area and the latest hearing device technology. As an independent, internationally regarded master of audiology, I trust his advice implicitly. ~**Brian James**

Luckily for me I heard a family friend singing Andrew's praises about his success in relation to hearing loss, so I contacted his clinic for an appointment. I can now say it was the best decision I could have made. My advice to anyone who has hearing loss is to contact an audiology professional. As for me, I was so lucky to have found Andrew Campbell. He and his team are definitely the professionals in this field, and it is with great confidence that I recommend him and his team. ~**Judith Cush**

We heard that Andrew was an independent audiologist and therefore free to prescribe whatever he thinks is suitable for each of his patients. The whole experience has been a revelation. Andrew quickly determined my hearing issues during that first appointment, and recommended very neat and discreet hearing aids. They were life-enhancing right from the start. I would recommend Andrew without hesitation as a caring, extremely knowledgeable professional who works with you to obtain the best results possible. ~**Gary James**

My mother was profoundly deaf for most of her life, and my two sisters and I all have a hearing loss, so we've been in the hearing space for a long time. I say this to put my comments on Andrew in context—he truly is a totally genuine, caring and fantastic audiologist. After attending one of his public lectures, which I thoroughly recommend, my sister and I decided to visit his clinic. We were both struggling with hearing in our respective workplaces. Andrew was able to find customized solutions for us that have been brilliant. He is extremely capable, knowledgeable, really listens to your concerns and is very patient when it comes to helping you with the technology side of things. We only wish we'd discovered him sooner. **~Nicole Price**

Hi Andrew, great session today and quite a few people have given very positive feedback to us about your Hearing and Brain Health seminar. Many, many thanks! **~U3A Deepdene Administration**

Published in Australia by
The Hearing and Brain Health Academy
PO Box 785
New Farm QLD 4005
1300 418 852
info@neuaudio.com.au
www.neuaudio.com.au

First published in Australia 2022
Copyright © Andrew Campbell 2022

National Library of Australia Cataloguing in Publication entry

 A catalogue record for this book is available from the National Library of Australia

ISBN: 978-0-6452598-4-1 (paperback)
ISBN: 978-0-6452598-5-8 (hardback)
ISBN: 978-0-6452598-7-2 (ebook)

Book designed by Sophie White
Printed by Ingram Spark

Disclaimer: This book offers health and lifestyle advice and is designed for educational purposes only. You should not rely on this information as a substitute for professional health and medical advice. If you have any health concerns, consult with a health care professional. Don't disregard or delay having medical health care advice from your health care professional because of what you have read in this book.

Hearing & Brain Health

Startling links between untreated hearing loss and cognitive decline

Andrew Campbell

Bac Soc Sci (Psych), MClinAud, MACAud

*To the scientific researchers
whose comprehensive work
helped inform this book.*

*May your efforts inspire those
living with untreated hearing
loss to take steps towards
a life without limitation.*

ABOUT THE AUTHOR

Andrew Campbell is a Masters trained, independent adult rehabilitation specialist audiologist, and a pioneer in the field of cognitive health and hearing. His passion is to help patients return to a fuller participation in life.

As a leader in hearing health care and audiological sciences, Andrew takes a holistic approach to hearing health. He inspires audiences across the world to address their hearing issues to protect the brain and to allow them to live flourishing lives without limitation.

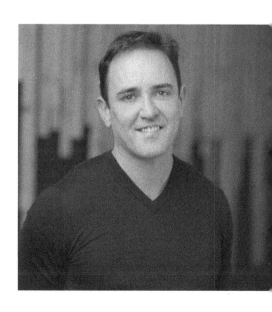

CONTENTS

FOREWORD

I was spurred into action when I heard Andrew Campbell speak about the impact of hearing loss on brain health. The fact that most concerned me was that hearing loss has been demonstrated to be the number one modifiable risk factor for dementia.

As a writer, words are my business and I had started to lose some of them. What was the word for that thing that you take out the rubbish in? It's green and smells a bit. It's on the tip of my tongue… The bin! Then of course the TV volume had crept up to neighbors-complaining volume and the subtitles were employed because all the actors mumbled. But still, I didn't book into an audiologist.

Yes, I'm one of those statistics—one of the one in ten who failed to do anything about my growing deafness. After reading *Hearing and Brain Health – Startling links between untreated hearing loss and cognitive decline*, I now understand the full consequences of not taking action. Why did I leave it? Because I was relatively young—in my fifties— and did not like the idea of wearing hearing aids. Then a friend told me about Andrew Campbell and suggested I go to one of his seminars. His presentation was eye-opening, and with some degree of trepidation on returning home I emailed him immediately for an appointment.

The whole experience changed my life. Now I can hear well, my hearing aids are barely detectable, and after six months of full-time use the words I was losing have nestled back into their rightful spots in my brain—the word 'bin' is readily available as and when I need it.

Hearing loss is one of the most undertreated medical conditions, which can and does have enormous impact on every aspect of our lives and health, and it is one of the easiest conditions to treat. Andrew Campbell has devoted his career to disseminating the message that people should deal with their hearing loss as early as possible to reduce the risk of cognitive decline and retain full participation in life.

As a pioneer in the field of hearing and brain health, Andrew presents compelling research that shows that dealing with health issues in isolation will not yield the best results. For instance, you may need to treat a clogged heart with surgery, but you would also be wise to address what caused the clogging in the first place—lifestyle, stresses, diet. Likewise, the hearing center of the brain also houses the memory and other cognitive functions, and the stress of hearing loss affects those other functions.

It's my fervent belief that *Hearing and Brain Health* is not just useful to people who experience hearing loss, it's a book that everyone can benefit from because fundamentally, it's about prevention of illness. At a basic level, hearing loss can isolate us from others and life. Untreated, it can cause us to withdraw because we cannot carry on a coherent conversation or hear in crowded environments. Science shows us that the stress of social isolation can be as deadly as the worst lifestyle habits, for instance, puffing on a pack of cigarettes a day, and studies show that elderly people who are bereft of social interaction are twice as likely to die prematurely.

I have no doubt that Andrew has and will continue to have an enormous impact on people's lives through his work. *Hearing and Brain Health* provides a wealth of accessible information about every aspect of treatable hearing issues. It's also very reassuring to read that the brain is plastic and much lost functionality may be restored by the simple act of wearing hearing aids for 12 or more hours a day. I am living proof of that. In his second book, *Your Resilient Brain*, he teaches us about taking a holistic approach to hearing loss, which includes strategies for enhancing overall mental capacity and function, and general health.

Janie Tzara

Introduction

Groundbreaking research conducted throughout the last decade reveals that hearing loss is the number one modifiable risk factor for dementia. How do the two afflictions relate to each other? It's simple. Hearing and memory are intimately intertwined in adjacent areas in the brain, and it's been proven that the strain of not being able to hear sufficiently affects the memory centers.

If you suffer hearing loss, this knowledge may cause concern, however, there's a good ending to the story. You're going to hear the words 'neuroplasticity' and 'cognitive function' quite a lot throughout this book. Research has shown clear links between untreated hearing loss and impaired cognitive function and that it's never too late to reduce your risk of cognitive decline and improve your quality of life.

In the western world people generally put off visiting a hearing specialist for between 7-10 years which, the science suggests, is 7-10 years too late for optimal outcomes. It's a strange phenomenon because we don't hesitate to go to an eye specialist when our eyesight is deteriorating, but we will find ways to compensate for hearing loss rather than see an audiologist.

Neglecting our hearing is damaging to our health in a myriad of ways. Over the course of the next 10–20 years, the proportion of people aged over 65 is expected to more than double; with this comes increasing ill health. When considering the unprecedented decline in fertility rates since the 1970s, there's also the added burden of having relatively fewer working-age people available to support sick and elderly people.

Ageing is more or less inevitable, but decline is optional. Whilst there's no cure for many common chronic conditions, treatments are becoming more effective, especially when they're delivered in time.

Associate Professor Daniel R George, from Penn State Hershey Medical Center and Penn State College of Medicine and Alzheimer's, states in an article, *Overcoming the social death of dementia through language*, "Alzheimer's disease is personified as a 'mind-robber' that 'attacks' or 'strikes' the brains of individuals, leaving plaques and tangles in its wake." No one finds the thought of that appealing.

Imagine for a moment that every person in your city or town woke up this morning at the age of 85. According to today's statistics, roughly 50 percent would have Alzheimer's disease—the most common form of dementia. The other 50 percent would need to essentially be fulltime caregivers of those with this dreadful disease. Imagine what the prevailing mood would be. What if during those preceding decades of incubation, something could have been done to prevent or moderate the development of Alzheimer's?

This example was used by renowned neuroscientist, Lisa Genova, in a TED talk presentation on Alzheimer's prevention in 2017. Her overall message was not one of doom and gloom - far from it. The talk offered a message of hope in the form of practical, straightforward, scientifically proven advice directed toward prevention. That's the form this book will take.

Lisa's talk, and dozens of scientific research papers, have informed this work. A silver-bullet cure for dementia doesn't exist, nor is there a cure for ageing or noise-related hearing loss. However, there are treatments and strategies that can substantially reduce their impact, and significantly improve a person's quality of life.

In addition, new research shows that our brains can change at any age, so there's plenty of hope. Most of the breakthroughs I'll discuss have only emerged over the past 10 years - and some are only months old. The neurosciences are now adding so much value that it's challenging to keep up. But as an avid researcher and Master of Audiology with training in the neurosciences, I bear good news. The future is bright.

I assume you've picked up this book as a proactive measure, and for that I tip my hat to you. It will give you an earful of educational research about the treatment of hearing loss with a focus on brain health. This approach is fresh and new in the auditory specialist profession, and it aims to make a big difference to broader aspects of your wellbeing and health.

Generally, I find that my patients are more concerned about cognitive decline than the nuisance of hearing loss. To paraphrase philosopher and neuroscientist Sam Harris: your mind is the basis of every experience you have and of every contribution you make to the lives of others. Given this fact, it makes sense to protect it.

The most common form of hearing loss is acquired later in life, and is essentially a progressive, degenerative disorder with neurological involvement. That simply means your hearing will continue to degrade as you age. It's genetically predetermined, and unless you're the recipient of a favorable mutation, it will happen to you if you live long enough. That's just the way it is. It can't be cured, but it can be treated.

As your doctor will tell you, just as with any other major chronic disorder, be it diabetes, cancer or coronary heart disease, there's immense value in catching and treating these conditions early. It's the same for hearing loss.

Much of what is considered health care in this day and age could better be described as 'sick care'. Little attention is paid to real prevention. The medical profession tends to talk about prevention as screening. I'm all about treating hearing loss when there's a possibility of restoring what has been lost and preserving residual functionality over the long term. The goal is to allow people to retain the faculties to live a full life.

All of this becomes more challenging the longer the

hearing centers in the brain have been deprived of stimulation. This is usually associated with decay of the auditory nerve. Recent neuroscience research highlights the urgency and importance of hearing loss treatment. New research published in *The Lancet* neurology journal found that changes in the brain and body occur up to 20 years before symptoms of the most common forms of dementia arise. This highlights the importance of a proactive approach.

Whilst there's no cure for dementia, measures can be taken to reduce its impact and slow its progression. Treating hearing loss is a straightforward, rapid intervention that supports brain health and quality of life. To this day, I've never fully understood the relative lack of importance people tend to place on addressing hearing loss, possibly because I've witnessed first-hand how simple and effective treatment is. However, I've found that once people are educated about what can be achieved, they see the enormous difference the simple solution of hearing aids can make to their quality of life.

Since I started publicly delivering this form of educational content over three years ago, not a day has gone by without a seminar attendee, book recipient or patient reaching out with gratitude for the newly acquired clarity about this insidious affliction. It seems there's a real thirst for insight into what is a daily struggle for millions. I can't think of a better contribution I can personally make to society than to articulate these messages and inspire others to pass it on, so please feel free to pay this book forward.

Broadly, *Hearing and Brain Health* will begin with the 'micro' physiological aspects of hearing loss and move to the 'macro' or broader impacts, including the impact it has on people who care about you.

To be well informed is to be well armed to hear life at its fullest. I truly hope you find it helpful.

PART 1

Emerge From Silence

CHAPTER 1

Hearing loss is awful, treatment is not

Right now, around one in ten people in the western world are living with untreated hearing loss. It could be the Uber driver that needs to look in the rear-view mirror to lip-read the passenger's directions, the grandmother missing most of the vows at her grandchild's wedding, or the waiter approaching retirement age who's petrified that he might get an order wrong.

If you're not one of the one in ten, I can guarantee you know someone who is. Untreated hearing loss is a mind robber, and its misdeeds extend well beyond a few missed words and the nuisance of strained communication.

Over my 20 years' experience as an audiologist, not a week has gone by without being confronted by the heartbreaking cases of those who left it too late. Take Madame Woo, a patient at my Malaysian practice, who believed the unfortunate myth prevalent in Asia at the time that hearing loss only needed to be treated when the person was nearly completely deaf. At the time I encountered her, she was a widow and unable to communicate with her children. On top of that, she was illiterate, having never learned to write.

Another one of my patients was Mrs. De Silva, who lived in a retirement community. The management called me in because of complaints about her blaring TV and the shouting that came from her room whenever her family came to visit.

Then there was Mr. Jones, a war veteran who lost most of his hearing due to frequent exposure to noisy aircrafts. His hearing loss and constant tinnitus (ringing in the ears) impacted nearly every aspect of his life and most notably was responsible for the strained relationship with his wife.

The list goes on.

The shouting would be comical if it weren't so devastating. These people put off treating their hearing loss for over a decade and consequently, were a challenge to treat. Moderate outcomes were possible but not the clarity in hearing that would have been achievable had they acted sooner.

How is it that an extremely common, highly treatable, yet potentially devastating condition can be confined to the shadows and frequently ignored? One reason is that hearing aids have somewhat of an image problem.

People tend to have outdated, preconceived attitudes toward hearing loss and hearing aids and are not aware of the modern solutions available today. So, it's important to address the predominant stigmas and misconceptions head-on.

Bone hard yet deeply sensitive

The most common causes of hearing loss are age and over-exposure to noise. These factors are responsible for what we audiologists call sensorineural hearing loss, which is a permanent, progressive, degenerative disorder with neurologic involvement.

In the case of older adults, around 80 percent experience some level of hearing loss, with a noise-induced component in around half of those cases. In situations where both ageing and noise exposure are factors, they combine to cause a relatively rapid decline. Noise exposure is very much likened to premature ageing of the hearing system; it simply speeds up the process.

The cochlea, which is the organ of hearing, has a finite number of receptor cells at the nerve endings that lead to the brain. These are referred to as inner and outer hair cells. The cochlea is roughly the size of a pea and contains around 15,000 hair cells. We have a cochlea in each ear, so we have around 30,000 hair cells in total.

Hair cells are the ear's equivalent to the rods and cones of the eye; they receive stimulation from external sounds and pass along the information as a complex series of electrically charged neurochemical signals to the brain's hearing centers.

The final number of hair cells is reached very early in our development (around 10 weeks of gestation); after this stage our cochlea can only lose hair cells.

The cochlea is deeply embedded in the skull, within the hardest bone in the body. It seems likely that it's so heavily protected as it's supremely important.

Imperfect pitch

We're genetically predetermined, as we age, to encounter hearing loss in a progressive and degenerative fashion. With this progressive degenerative disorder, comes the gradual, continual damage and loss of hair cells within the cochlea. Most hair cells have approximately 30 nerve fibers responsible for relaying information to the brain to process sounds, conversation, music and so on. They also play a role in selectively suppressing and enhancing certain sounds in challenging listening situations.

The most delicate hair cells are the ones that are stimulated by high-pitched sounds. Like the high-pitched strings of a guitar, violin, or piano, high-pitch hair cells are thin, fine, and break more easily. Consequently, people most commonly first lose their hearing in the high pitches. This often means they miss the higher-pitched consonants that generally contain the meaning of words. This happens as each cell dies, along with the attached neurons.

Recent research indicates we only find a loss of sensitivity in the audiogram (the most common hearing assessment) when around 50 percent or more of those 30 nerve fibers attached to each of the most common hair cells are lost. Whilst the audiogram is an important clinical tool that tells us quite a lot, it is a relatively blunt instrument that does not always capture the true impact hearing loss has on one's quality of life. There's a relatively high degree of individual variability, much of which is determined by how long hearing loss has been left untreated.

Damage to the hair cells is irreversible; however, the neural pathways in the brain, beyond the hair cells, are 'plastic', which means they can be strengthened, and new connections can be formed. What happens beyond the ear, with reference to the neural pathways in the brain, is most interesting because it has the potential to be restimulated and restrengthened. To do that, we first need to overcome the barrier or hurdle created by the weakening of the inner ear. Put simply, hearing aids, worn consistently, treat the brain by overcoming the obstacle of hearing loss. However, the longer these neural connections are left under-stimulated, the higher the likelihood of neural decay and auditory deprivation in the brain, which means it's more of a challenge to return them to full strength.

Generally, vowels are louder in volume and lower in pitch or tone than consonants, and therefore less affected when it comes to this loss in the higher frequencies. The consonants, however, are softer in volume and higher in pitch or tone than the vowels. They generally give us the clear meaning of words, which is why comprehension can suffer when this type of hearing loss occurs. Loss of high-frequency hearing usually occurs so gradually that people are often unaware it's happening. They tend to dismiss their inability to hear properly, believing that others are mumbling or not articulating their words.

CHAPTER 2

Fading into the background

High-pitch hearing loss makes it difficult to hear in background noise. There are several reasons for this. At a basic level, people with a high pitch hearing loss generally rely heavily on their low pitch hearing to follow conversation. Background noise, however, tends to be primarily lower in pitch, which can impact the clarity of low pitch speech content. The lower the pitch, the longer the wavelength. These sounds are better able to bend around objects and travel distances than high-pitch sounds. The result is that the lower pitch vowels and consonants that are often critical for speech understanding are often masked out by background noise.

In noisy situations, people with normal hearing tend to rely on their ability to hear high-frequency consonant sounds to follow a conversation. People with high-pitch hearing loss find it more challenging to hear the consonants, which makes it harder to follow conversations in noise, especially when the speaker's face can't be seen for lipreading and facial cues.

Visual cues are hugely important, but they're not always possible. Hearing and understanding full words from another room, from behind facemasks or where a speaker's face can't be seen, for instance in TV programs and movies, can be exceptionally challenging.

Reliance on vision becomes more important for the hearing impaired. As parts of words (most commonly consonants) are increasingly missed, use of visual cues such as body language, facial expressions and lip movements become increasingly important for communication. But that can come at a cost.

In early 2020, researchers at the University of Maryland demonstrated that even in cases of mild levels of hearing loss, visual centers of the brain started to encroach on the hearing centers. This process is called cross-modal reorganization, and the researchers found it occurs within six months of acquiring hearing loss. According to the research, the downsides of such reorganization are that hearing in background noise becomes more challenging, and cognitive impairments emerge, such as short-term memory loss, which slows the brain's processing speed and impairs executive function. Executive function refers to overarching mental processes such as self-control, emotional regulation, and the ability to plan, focus, and remember instructions.

The good news is that cross-modal reorganization and the associated deficits were shown to be reversible with consistent use of quality hearing devices over a six-month period. Via MRI imagery, functional, and electrophysiological tests, researchers were able to demonstrate that the hearing centers returned to a better condition. The auditory cortex, which is part of the brain that plays a critical role in perceiving sound, was shown to be more intact and performing its role more directly. Prior to hearing aid fitting, the auditory cortex had actually reorganized away from where it is normally located in the brain. Hearing in background noise also improved, as did performance on a range of cognitive tests.

Our brains play a critical role in focusing on and separating out sounds. Hearing loss can stifle this function. Our ability to recognize certain sounds and voices occurs in the brain. Have you ever noticed that in a noisy room, you can pick up when your name is spoken, even if other words aren't clear? This is because a complex interaction occurs between your ears, your memory, and the filters your brain applies to wanted and unwanted sounds. The ability to focus on certain sounds and separate them from others, such as hearing a person at a cocktail party amongst other speakers and noise, requires complex processing.

The outer hair cells, which are at the end of nerves that are most susceptible to damage through ageing and noise exposure, play an important part in the focusing and separation processes. In complex listening situations, an intricate process takes place between the ears. The outer hair cells help us selectively filter out unwanted sounds. When those outer hair cells are damaged, their function becomes limited, making hearing in background noise more challenging.

According to the World Health Organization (WHO), hearing impairment affects around 1.5 billion people worldwide. On top of this, dementia cases are predicted to triple over the next few decades. However, considering the findings of a recently published study (July 2021) in *Alzheimer's & Dementia:*

The Journal of the Alzheimer's Association, the dementia statistics may also be influenced by our capacity to understand speech in noise.

Researchers at the University of Oxford's Nuffield Department of Population Health investigated the links between Alzheimer's disease and hearing loss in the largest study of its kind. They discovered that when people found it hard to hear spoken conversation in the presence of background noise, they had up to a 91 percent increased risk of developing dementia.

In the study, a group of 82,000 women and men aged 60 or older were tested over an 11-year period to assess their capacity to hear speech-in-noise (the ability to hear in noisy situations). During the 11 years, 1,285 participants were identified as developing dementia based on hospital inpatient and death register records. The study demonstrated that "insufficient" or "poor" speech-in-noise hearing, as determined by the study criteria, were associated with a 61 percent and 91 percent increased risk of developing dementia respectively, compared to normal speech-in-noise hearing.

Treating speech-in-noise hearing impairment may

be a promising intervention for dementia prevention, especially given that difficulties with hearing in background noise is one of the most common symptoms associated with age-related hearing loss.

UK Alzheimer's Researcher, Dr. Katy Stubbs commented on the Oxford study, stating that, "While most people think of memory problems when we hear the word dementia, this is far from the whole story. Many people with dementia will experience difficultly following speech in a noisy environment—a symptom sometimes called the 'cocktail party problem'. This study suggests that these hearing changes may not just be a symptom of dementia, but a risk factor that could potentially be treated."

Due to advances in hearing aid technology, modern hearing aids can "separate" noise, and focus on the desired sounds to supplement the weakened hearing processes of a damaged auditory system. In the past three years, numerous new solutions have emerged, making hearing in background noise even easier.

Several years ago, patients used to complain because their hearing devices actually increased the levels of background noise. This was true for many of the older style of devices. However, many modern hearing aids now have the capability for binaural beamforming, which allows the microphones to work together as a team. This is a binaural ability, meaning that it involves both of the ears and it improves hearing in background noise. With binaural beamforming, research indicates a person is around 30 percent more likely to understand speech in background noise compared to hearing aids that don't have that capability. In fact, several studies have shown that binaural beamforming technology can even give wearers an advantage over people with normal hearing, provided their hearing loss is in the mild to moderate range.

This is not to suggest that the ultimate replacement part exists. Even the most advanced solutions require a period of adaptation and consistent daily use to be effective in challenging listening environments. There are literally thousands of adjustments that can be made, so it's important that the devices are correctly customized by an experienced clinician. The most important thing to remember, which is a key to overall hearing and cognitive health success, is that you actually have to wear the hearing aids for between 12-16 hours a day.

CHAPTER 3

Flexible mind, flexible brain

For centuries, the brain was believed to be hardwired like a piece of machinery and utterly immutable. This belief has been disproven. The brain is constantly changing and has the ability to rewrite its future. This phenomenon is called neuroplasticity, or put simply, the capacity for the brain to change.

Neuroplasticity is a dynamic set of processes that can occur at any age. Until recently, it was assumed the brain was a static organ that reached its growth potential at around age 17. In the 1990s, ground-breaking research demonstrated significant changes in the brains of older adults as a result of learning. This sparked further interest and research on the ongoing ability for our brains to change.

Neuroplasticity happens in adults
in three main ways:

1. Forming new connections

Every time you learn something new, you form new connections, which happens at any age. The exciting phenomenon of neuroplasticity generally occurs in adults via the creation of new connections between existing neurons.

2. Strengthening existing connections

Every time you repeat an activity or practice a skill, the associated pathways strengthen. Over time, myelin—a fatty, gray-looking substance—grows around frequently used neural fibers, improving the strength and speed of the brain's electrical signals.

3. Removing or reducing unused pathways

A process known as pruning occurs in parts of the brain that are no longer stimulated, such as the neural pathways connected to damaged nerve endings in the inner ear. Put simply, use it or lose it.

The key message is that not all damage or loss of connections are set in stone - your brain can change for the better at any age.

Hearing aids can facilitate favorable neuroplasticity

The revelation of the connection between hearing loss and cognitive decline first came to light in 2011 when Dr. Frank Lin, from the Johns Hopkins Medical Centre, published a major longitudinal study on ageing. In his study, over 600 participants aged around 60 came to the center for two to three days a year for testing over a 12-year period. None of the participants had dementia at the commencement of this research.

The researchers assessed a range of factors associated with ageing. Hearing loss was just one of those factors, and it was not the core focus of the study.

Above all other findings of the study, the most remarkable and surprising were the clear links between untreated hearing loss and dementia. An increased dementia risk correlated clearly with the degree of hearing loss.

Researchers demonstrated a 200 percent increased risk of dementia at mild levels of hearing loss (around a 20-40% loss), 300 percent at moderate levels (around a 40-60% loss) and 500 percent at severe levels (around a 60% loss or more).

Further investigation found that hearing loss was associated with an acceleration of cognitive decline by 30-40 percent. This equates to a premature ageing of cognitive abilities by on average 6.8 years for every 25dB (roughly 25%) of hearing loss. This would suggest that, on average, a 66-year-old with a 50 percent untreated hearing loss would have the approximate brain age of an 80-year-old.

With all this in mind, shouldn't hearing loss be the first thing we consider when our faculties begin to fade?

It's important to note that such significant and concerning findings are peer reviewed and robust. I had the pleasure and privilege of attending intensive training by Professor Frank Lin, and he indicated that such findings have been repeated with remarkable reliability in separate studies by other universities.

Prof. Lin's impressive work sparked a lot of additional research into this important field and was central in informing landmark reports published in *The Lancet*, a renowned medical journal. In December 2017, *The Lancet* published a major article demonstrating that hearing loss was the number one modifiable risk factor for the prevention of dementia — 'modifiable' meaning that you can do something about it.

In an extensive review, the European Council for Dementia Prevention concluded that based on the best peer reviewed research, 35 percent of dementia cases could be prevented. The strongest intervention they found was treating hearing loss at middle age. They also reported that social isolation, depression, and low physical activity were important factors in relation to untreated hearing loss.[1] These factors, combined, account for over half of the modifiable lifestyle factors reported in the study.

Many of these studies were included in a 2020 update of the 2017 Lancet paper.[1]

The following is a summary of three major studies on the protective role of hearing devices for cognitive health.

- A 25-year study of 3,777 people aged 65 years or older found an increased dementia incidence in those with self-reported hearing problems *except* in those using hearing aids.

- A 2018 cross–sectional study in the UK of 7,385 people found that hearing loss was only

1   Research references listed in the appendices.

associated with worse cognition in those with untreated hearing loss (those not using hearing aids).

- A survey of 2,040 people older than 50 years in the United States, who were tested every two years for 18 years, found that memory recall deteriorated less after initiating hearing aid use. Hearing aid use was shown to be the largest factor protecting people from decline in memory recall.

This is great news! It's important to note that although the researchers in these studies indicated that full-time use (at least 12 hours per day) of hearing devices was difficult to control in such studies, the evidence suggests that full-time use would reinforce these significant findings.

One study that required consistent 12-plus hours per day of hearing device use demonstrated both functional and structural improvements in the brain over a 12-month period. This study, titled 'Anatomical and Functional MRI Changes after One Year of Auditory Rehabilitation with Hearing Aids' (a typically snappy name for a scientific study!) was published in *Neural Plasticity Journal* in 2018. Functional MRI images were taken of 14 people's brains prior to hearing device use. The researchers monitored the regularity of use over a year, and then reassessed those same areas of the brain with imaging and functional assessments. They found that not only did the hearing centers in the brain function better, there was also a significant increase in the physical size of these centers.

Studies show that hearing aids perform better than any dementia drugs

On top of that, hearing aids have been shown to be twice as effective as the best available drugs in preventing cognitive decline.

Following the review of a recent study comparing the best dementia prevention drugs and the treatment of hearing loss in the fight for dementia prevention, Dr. Murali Doraiswamy M.D., a professor of psychiatry and medicine at Duke University School of Medicine and co-author of *The Alzheimer's Action Plan* concluded: "The benefits of correcting hearing loss on cognition are twice as large as the benefits from any cognitive-enhancing drugs now on the market. It should be the first thing we focus on."

That's quite a profound statement, considering the billions of pharmaceutical research dollars spent on this mind-robbing disease.

Nobel Prize winning neurologist, Erik Kandel, is also an advocate for treating hearing loss for cognitive benefit. He recommends annual hearing evaluations and hearing device use, because hearing aids provide brain training with relatively immediate results. He reports significant increases in selective attention, memory recall and processing speed just two weeks post-hearing aid fitting.

Clearly, hearing loss has serious neurological consequences.

Kindness is the language which the deaf can hear and the blind can see.

~Mark Twain

CHAPTER 4

Lifestyle issues and mechanisms linked to cognitive decline

The big picture around cognitive decline and hearing loss is multi-factorial, but hearing aids are a significant benefit for a variety of reasons. The best research I can find focuses on three main mechanisms: social isolation, cognitive overload, and cerebral atrophy.

Worlds apart

As hearing in noisy situations becomes more challenging, people tend to avoid being social. Not only is it exhausting trying to hear someone talk while there's background noise, it can also potentially be humiliating. You could be nodding and smiling when someone delivers bad news. You could answer what you thought was a question but was really a statement or miss the punchline of a joke. "I'll pick you up in an hour," could be heard as "you need a shower." These situations can be very tricky.

Unfortunately, a common trend is to stay at home and avoid such situations. This is the point where your world becomes smaller, and you're doing less of the things you once enjoyed.

Social isolation, in this context, does not just refer to the avoidance of parties, clubs and bars. Hearing loss frequently has domestic, 'at home' implications. As communication becomes more challenging, there can be a tendency to stick to the basics. Nuance, humor, intimacy, and even close relationships can become stifled, as it becomes increasingly hard to communicate effectively. This is not only isolating for the hearing-impaired person, but for anyone else in the conversation.

Then come the least favored, or dare I say disliked responses, to those who cannot hear well, such as 'never mind' or 'it doesn't matter'. This kind of dismissive communication can be incredibly isolating, not to mention infuriating over the long-term.

Social isolation and loneliness can have far-reaching consequences. Studies have shown strong links to depression, anxiety, and reduced physical activity. Recent research by the Centers for Disease Control and Prevention indicates that loneliness can increase dementia risk by 50 percent and increase the risk of premature death by 45 percent. There are also strong links between loneliness and coronary heart disease, which equates to the approximate health effects of smoking 15 cigarettes per day.

Feeling isolated and lonely is stressful. Studies show that lonely people have higher levels of the stress hormone, cortisol, and are consequently at a high risk of developing a variety of chronic diseases. As the saying goes, a problem shared is a problem halved. By treating your hearing loss, you're better able to engage with others, maintain relationships, and stay sharp in social, family, community, and work situations while maintaining social supports to handle life's challenges.

Cognitive overload

Since the advent of modern agriculture around 10,000 years ago, not much has changed or evolved in the physical structure of our hearing system. This has been confirmed through examination of the remains of the ancients. People didn't live much beyond the age of 30 at that time, and the loudest sounds were likely to be the occasional shout or thunderclap.

Age-related and noise-induced hearing loss, which impact our ability to hear high-pitch consonants, were unlikely to be a feature of daily life back then. In fact, the phenomenon of high-pitch hearing loss was not formally recognized in medical literature until the late 1800s.

Given what we know about the recent emergence of the most common forms of hearing loss, the notion of supplementing the auditory parts of conversation with the visual parts (through lip reading) may well be described as a modern-day practice. It's not something we've evolved to be particularly good at, as evidenced by the measurable cognitive load that ensues, as well as the reorganization that occurs in the brain, that appears to impair our capacity to hear in background noise as well as our cognition.

Piecing together parts of words is a challenge for our ancient brains. Hearing loss is tiring and puts strain on the brain. Research tells us that the more unclear words are and the more listening effort that is required to hear them, the less likely those words are going to be remembered. The process of lipreading requires a complex interaction between vision, hearing, and short- and long-term memory. It can be exhausting and taxing on our limited cognitive resources, as highlighted in the cross-modal reorganization studies outlined earlier. One of my patients described it aptly: "It's like going 100kms per hour in second gear".

Researchers theorize that the 'always on' strain on the brain associated with untreated hearing loss over the long-term is a contributing factor to heightened dementia risk and memory impairment.

Turn the volume up

Cerebral atrophy (brain shrinkage) is associated with under-stimulation of the brain. Untreated hearing loss has been shown to result in up to a 40 percent volume loss in parts of the brain associated with memory, language, speech, and hearing. The neural pathways in the brain are, in some respects, like muscles—if you don't use them, they reduce in size and function. With limited stimulation over time (studies indicate 10 years or more), the deterioration of the neural connections between the ears and brain may be permanent.

To overcome the barrier presented by damaged nerve endings, hearing aids provide proper stimulation and exercise to the 'plastic' hearing centers in the brain, thereby reducing cognitive load and listening effort and enabling a return to a fuller participation in life.

Sound Employment, Engagement & Economics

Since 1989, Sergei Kochkin at the Better Hearing Institute has conducted large scale research on the hearing aid market. One such major study focused on the correlation between hearing loss and earning potential. This study indicated that untreated hearing loss could reduce annual earnings by as much as $30,000 per annum. However, when hearing aids were worn consistently, the risk of decreased earnings was reduced by up to 90 percent. The core explanation is that effective verbal communication is required for higher levels of responsibility. Overall quality of life improvement needs to be taken into account here too, because consistently worn hearing devices help reduce the negative impacts associated with untreated hearing loss. This includes anxiety, depression, social isolation, social paranoia, emotional stability, and cognitive functioning.

Many of my patients have retired from regular employment, yet are actively involved with community groups, busy with family commitments, or engaged with ongoing education. These activities give people a sense of purpose, meaning and dignity later in life, so it's paramount to sustain them. It's somewhat of a challenge to put a dollar figure on that, especially when we consider that untreated hearing loss doesn't just impact the person, but those who interact *with* them. When communication is clear and effortless, without the burden of hearing loss, such an intervention is highly valuable.

In 2019, Robert Brent, Professor of Economics at Fordham University, published a cost-benefit analysis of treating hearing loss. This analysis considered recent statistics regarding cognitive factors, quality of life, and earning potential. In a series of complicated and well researched equations, he concluded that the total benefits of treating hearing loss relative to the cost was extremely large, with a cost benefit ratio of over 30 to 1. This is to say that for every $1 spent on hearing loss treatment, there was more than a $30 pay off - most of these being direct benefits.

There's no doubt about it, hearing aids can be expensive. But I'd argue that there's a greater cost to doing nothing or taking a half measure, such as buying cheap, inadequate devices. Substandard devices tend not to be worn often because they may lack the ability to achieve effective outcomes and properly address a person's hearing needs. Research shows that hearing aids need to be worn consistently to achieve the full benefits. In my view, solutions need to be comfortable and effective enough to be worn at least 12 hours per day. It's concerning when suboptimal hearing solutions are chosen, because this may result in inadequate wear-time and therefore insufficient cognitive impacts, under-stimulation of the critical hearing centers of the brain, and social implications.

CHAPTER 5

Blindness vs deafness

Would you rather be deaf or blind? Studies show that on average, when posed with this unthinkable hypothetical, 83 percent of people would prefer to be deaf when given the choice over blindness, and just 17 percent would prefer blindness over deafness. Given these findings, it's little wonder that people in the Western world are around five times more likely to treat vision loss. Those who state they would choose hearing over vision as a preference mainly cite aesthetic reasons for their preference. They want to be able to appreciate things such as music and the sounds of nature. Curiously, in such deafness vs blindness opinion polls, rarely is communication mentioned as an important facet of hearing. However, science tells us a different story.

In the 75-year-long happiness study at Harvard University, researchers found that happiness was a clear result of quality relationships and that the happiest people were that way because of the quality of their closest relationships. There's no question that effective communication and the ability to hear clearly is crucial in maintaining our closest relationships. The study found that the least happy people were lonely. Lonely people were shown to have reduced brain volumes, shorter lifespans, and were more likely to be depressed.

You may have heard of "Blue Zones" - regions in the world where people are significantly more likely to reach ages over 100 years old. These zones, situated in Ikaria in Greece, Okinawa in Japan, the Ogliastra region in Sardinia, Loma Linda in California, and the Nicoya Peninsula in Costa Rica, are of supreme interest to researchers, public health officials, and the medical community.

Psychologist Susan Pinker describes one of the Blue Zone studies in her book, *The Village Effect*. One curious finding takes place on the island of Sardinia. Not only were inhabitants more likely to live over 100 years of age than people living elsewhere, but it was the only place with no difference in the life expectancy between men and women. In the other Blue Zones, and in much of the Western world, women typically outlive men by approximately seven years. But not in Sardinia. When examining the habits and priorities of Sardinian men, the researchers could find no clear difference in how men and women prioritized relationships. In fact, Sardinian men were equally likely to invest time in their families and close friendships as women, which is not always the case for men in the rest of the world. Large scale, multivariate psychological studies indicate that in general, men have a proclivity for 'things', and women have a proclivity for 'people'. It seems, as found in the Harvard study, that orienting to people through quality relationships may be central in securing a longer, happier life.

Imagine that you have a miniature fruit tree in the middle of your brain. This tree thrives on quality relationships, and provides the fruits which nourish your body and brain with positive emotion, vitality, and longevity. Where would this tree be drawing its sustenance? Which senses would be central to nourishing these quality relationships? If there were a superior or most important sense for relationship building, what would it be?

In thinking about the senses, communication, hearing, and relationships, a few examples come to mind from recent personal experiences. Over the COVID-19 crisis, Zoom meetings and video conferences became a daily reality of my work, family, and social life. Often there was an excruciating minute or two where the video would work but not the audio, and at times the audio wouldn't work at all. Beyond an awkward wave or smile, there really wasn't much that could be achieved during the interaction, let alone build the relationship.

Another example relates to my clinical practice. I occasionally see people who have lost their hearing completely. Recently, a patient who was dependent on one severely impaired ear, broke her device and couldn't hear at all. She and her husband were distraught, and communication in the clinic was limited to the painful to and fro process of writing notes. Such experiences can be agonizing.

Can you think of your own similar, silent experiences? Our relationship to communication can be akin to a fish's relationship to water. When it's always achievable, we tend not to notice it. In the Sardinian Blue Zones example, the researchers dug deep into men's orientation to relationships. Were they deliberately investing their time in people to prolong their lives? No. When questioned intensively it was revealed that's just how life was for these men.

Prioritizing relationships was the only way of life they knew.

Let's relate this back to people's tendency to value the aesthetic qualities of hearing, rather than the communication aspects. Could it be that when we're used to having it around, like fish in water, we tend to take it for granted and gasp for it only when it's out of reach?

In relative terms, complete deafness and complete blindness are exceptionally rare. Although, I find they do help to illustrate a point. In my experience, which the data supports, most people addressing a hearing loss for the first time have an approximate hearing loss of 20-40 percent, which is far from complete deafness. Not knowing the statistics in detail, I suspect that people addressing vision loss for the first time have a partial loss and are far from being completely blind. Although, I speculate that a partial hearing loss has a far greater impact on relationships with loved ones, whereas the frustration of a partial vision loss is almost completely confined to the individual.

When Helen Keller, the first deaf and blind person to achieve a university degree, was asked whether she'd prefer to keep her hearing or vision if given the choice, she, like others in her predicament, stated that she would hands down choose to have the ability to hear.

Don't wait until it's too late

Treating hearing loss is one of the most simple and effective ways of returning to a fuller participation in life, with additional benefits to overall health and wellbeing beyond hearing. The key to this is to catch it early and treat it early, just as you would with other chronic conditions such as heart disease, cancer, and diabetes.

As long as hearing loss is treated in its early stages and hearing devices are consistently worn, there's strong evidence of protection against associated cognitive decline, alongside the reversal of some of the detrimental impacts that hearing loss has on the brain.

Is treating hearing loss a 100 percent guarantee of lifelong dementia prevention? Sadly not, there's other factors to consider. But the evidence of its cognitive benefits is compelling, thorough, and continues to build.

*Blindness separates us from things;
deafness separates us from people.*

~Helen Keller

PART 2

The Nuts & Bolts

CHAPTER 6

Why hearing aids are relegated to the bathroom cabinet

People are five times more likely to wear their prescription glasses than their hearing aids. Why is it so? In my practice, I've noticed the following three trends:

One: Hearing aid owners simply weren't told to wear their devices every waking hour. Not a week goes by where I don't explain the benefits of full-time use to someone who has purchased their hearing aids elsewhere and seldom wears them. In fact, often times, it's literally as if it was their first time hearing this advice. Perhaps the audiologist who fitted the devices was under company-imposed time restraints (which is unfortunately common), or wasn't sufficiently educated in the benefits of full-time use to pass on this vital information.

I estimate that around 50 percent of my clinical

time is in some way related to ensuring that certain conditions are met so that my patients actually wear their devices. One of the great features of modern hearing aids is that their usage can be tracked by an audiologist through the databases built into all devices.

Two: The acclimatization period was incomplete. When hearing loss is finally treated, after a delay of somewhere between three to thirty years, there's a lot to get used to. It's an adaptive process. Like a muscle that hasn't been exercised, the neural pathways take time to strengthen.

The brain also needs to relearn to filter the useful sounds from those that are not. This process takes time.

For most people, 12-16 hours of use a day, over a period of 7-10 days at conservative settings does the trick. Sometimes further adjustment is needed. It's a personalized process, that depends on the degree of loss, how long the hearing loss has been around, personal sound preferences, and volume tolerance. The early stages are the most challenging in getting used to the devices. But with time and patience, everything tends to get better and feel more natural.

Three: Devices were uncomfortable for full-time use. If they're not comfortable, they simply won't be worn the way they need to be. Normally, in experienced hands, the physical fit can be improved substantially. Volume and noise reduction settings can also be adjusted in most cases, as long as the hearing device is sophisticated enough to allow for adjustment.

Sometimes people are concerned about the look of the devices. This is less of an issue these days, with the availability of much more inconspicuous and cosmetically pleasing options

Glasses half full

The hearing system is completely different to the visual one, so while reading glasses may effectively be used sporadically for reading, hearing aids should not only be used for conversation. The full benefits and value of hearing aids can only be experienced with full-time use. Glasses can assist with improving vision, a function which takes place in the eyes. In contrast, the ability to focus on what you want to hear occurs at the level of the brain, not at the ear. Wearing hearing devices on a part-time basis creates confusion, because it's challenging for the brain to constantly refocus when volume levels vary.

When hearing aids are only worn on a part-time basis, it's hard for the brain to know which sounds are helpful and which aren't. Whether it's the ticking of a clock, the whirring of the air conditioner or the humm of the refrigerator, some sounds are always present, but having our hearing focused on them serves no useful purpose. Ordinarily, you only really hear them when you listen out for them.

If you're wearing hearing devices for the first time, the brain needs to relearn where to apply the filters on helpful versus unhelpful sounds. This process takes time and is expedited when the hearing aids are worn full-time.

Inevitable changes to the way you hear your own voice also become more natural when you wear your devices full-time.

Don't fall for the hearing myth

Another benefit of full-time hearing aid use is the reduced risk of falls. Studies show that untreated hearing loss, even at mild levels, result in a 300 percent increased risk of falls for 40 to 69-year-olds. Researchers cite two main reasons for this. The first reason relates to environmental awareness. With untreated hearing loss, you're less likely to hear the sounds of things that may trip you up. This includes the sound of your feet on steps or a bike or scooter whizzing past.

The second reason relates to the sheer mental resources it takes to compensate for hearing loss, leaving less attention for steadiness and balance. Falls account for 25 percent of all hospital admissions and 40 percent of all nursing home admissions; 40 percent of those admitted do not return to independent living and 25 percent pass away within a year. As alarming as these statistics are, they are actually an underestimation, as many falls go unreported.

Separate to this, a major cause of falls in the elderly is when they get up to answer the phone. Some of the latest hearing aids integrate with mobile phones and are handsfree, so there's no need for elderly people to rush to answer the phone. Full-time hearing aid use helps to reduce the risk for hearing-related falls.

Today's hearing aids are modern marvels with apps and Bluetooth and the ability to make them comfortable in every way. It's vital to wear them for 12-16 hours per day. If comfort is an issue, let us or your audiologist know.

But what a humiliation for me when someone standing next to me heard a flute in the distance and I heard nothing, or someone standing next to me heard a shepherd singing and again I heard nothing. Such incidents drove me almost to despair; a little more of that and I would have ended my life—it was only my art that held me back.

~Ludwig van Beethoven

CHAPTER 7

The brain can be trained

Brain training can fast-track neural rewiring

Because a significant portion of our hearing processes take place in the brain where some of the memory centers sit, stress from the inability to hear can put strain on our cognitive abilities. Seeing an audiologist, getting your hearing loss treated, then wearing hearing aids for 12-16 hours a day will likely restore some of that impairment. Other easy interventions can also strengthen cognitive function.

Innovative brain training programs can improve cognitive function and speech in the presence of background noise. Depending on the program and length of training, improvements may also be seen in short term memory, as well as our ability to focus and sustain attention, process information, and react quickly. Each of these cognitive abilities can assist us in processing speech in challenging situations.

The best hearing specific program online training I've been able to find is called clEAR and is based on research performed by scientists working at Washington University in St. Louis. It's comprehensive, customizable, and delivered on an easy to navigate platform. It's the only auditory training program that allows you to train with a Frequent Communication Partner such as your spouse. Whilst the program is delivered in an American accent, the developers assure me it is just as effective for other accents. The training games in the program are designed to be enjoyable, so you may choose to play them even if they weren't good for you. Visit **clearworks4ears.com** to access further information about clEAR and the program itself.

There's also evidence that more general cognitive brain training programs can assist with dementia prevention over the long term. Undertaking such programs can be an ideal complement to hearing aid treatment and improve hearing in noisy environments. According to research conducted by the University of Western Australia, two programs, BrainHQ and Cognifit, provide the gold standard for online brain training. Following a review of the literature and my personal use of both programs, I tend to favor Cognifit because it has an objective score that you can improve over time via its personalized training program.

It's recommended that the personalized training program be done every second day for 15-20 minutes, and it's highly motivating to watch the score improve as you progress.

Check out **Cognifit.com** for more information.

A final word about brain training programs - they require a somewhat sustained commitment. I've found that over the past three years since I've been recommending them, people tend not to stick with them! Most programs take at least 3 months of consistent practice to be beneficial. Like other forms of fitness, brain training requires consistency over time to be effective.

If you would like further information about hearing and brain health, I've developed additional resources that may be of interest. In my second book, *Your Resilient Brain*, I present nine of the most impactful hearing and brain health interventions to protect and improve cognitive health, hearing, and general health and wellbeing. I've also developed a free, online, Hearing & Brain Health Academy. The course consists of eight videos where I present additional detail about the far-reaching impacts of untreated hearing loss, its effect on cognitive health, and the science and studies behind it.

https://neuaudio.link/brainhealth

CHAPTER 8

What to expect in your hearing evaluation appointment

Whether you're a first timer or accompanying a friend or family member to their hearing evaluation appointment, it's helpful and reassuring to know what to expect. Hearing tests are straightforward and simple, and most importantly, they are painless, non-invasive, and easy—no studying required!

It begins with taking a brief hearing history so we can investigate the potential cause of hearing loss and the impacts it may be having on your lifestyle and relationships. The ear canal is then inspected with a device called an otoscope. This is to check for physical problems that may block the free passage of sounds, such as earwax build-up or abnormal growths.

Following that, your hearing is assessed using various tests. These allow us to identify the root cause of any hearing issues. Hearing is a complex process. It begins with air vibrations (sound), which causes the ear drum to vibrate and send mechanical energy through the middle ear system. This mechanical energy is transduced into an electrochemical signal in the inner ear, leading to neural signals propagating throughout numerous structures in the brain.

There are three types of hearing tests that are conducted in a routine assessment:

One: Pure-tone audiometry

For this test, a variety of sounds of different pitches and volumes are played into headphones or insert earphones. You simply press a button each time you hear the sound. This allows us to chart what you can and can't hear.

Two: Speech recognition

The speech recognition test assesses your ability to distinguish words in the absence of visual cues like lip movements or facial expressions. During this test you're played words through headphones or earphones. This test reveals which aspects of speech that are not being heard due to hearing loss.

Three: Bone conduction assessment

This painless test involves a small vibrating headband placed against your skull and behind the ear. It measures how well sound, conducted through your skull, is detected by the inner ear. It also tests the efficiency of the inner ear and the associated auditory nerves.

Each test plays an important role in not only diagnosing hearing loss but determining the impact it may be having on your life. It helps us identify the most appropriate avenue for treatment. If we find a weakness in your hearing ability, we may conduct a hearing device demonstration and possibly a hearing device fitting. For this purpose, it can be exceptionally helpful if you are able to attend your appointment with someone who has a familiar voice. There can be quite a bit to take in. Many of our patients say that they find it useful to have another set of ears to support them.

The repercussions of hearing loss extend well beyond the person who has it. Whether you're seeing myself or another audiologist, having a loved one or two along for the assessment can often assist in determining the best course of action. Hearing is a family affair.

Hearing loss is often such a gradual phenomenon that the person is in denial. You really have to be patient with them in getting them to come forward for help.

~Marion Ross

CHAPTER 9

Common barriers & concerns

For most people, the prospect of taking the first step to treat hearing loss is daunting. Unlike a trip to the doctor or dentist, it's hard to know what to expect. Often there are essential questions people need to ask. However, many of them go unspoken. I call these 'the eight elephants in the room'.

Elephant #1: "I already know what the diagnosis will be."

If you've put off having a hearing assessment because you're reasonably sure of the likely outcome, you're not alone. At your appointment, you'll get the full picture of your hearing health. You'll also learn how simple the treatment can be.

Elephant #2: "Hearing aids look like big ugly beige bananas."

People with hearing loss in the 13th century used hollowed out cow or ram horns as hearing devices.

Much more sophisticated ear trumpets were invented in the 18th century. These didn't amplify sound. Instead, they "collected" the sound and funneled it through a narrow tube into the ear. The 20th century delivered the big beige banana transistors—the first behind-the-ear hearing aid. Fortunately, much has changed.

The last time I fitted a big beige banana was around 20 years ago and I still feel a bit embarrassed. Alas, that was what we had to work with at the time. Today's devices are modern and discreet. Most enable seamless interactivity with your smartphone and TV. There are completely invisible options too, although these may involve a trade-off in functionality. If hearing devices are warranted, rest assured that it won't be a big beige banana.

Elephant #3: "I don't want to draw attention to my hearing loss."

Whilst hearing loss itself is invisible, the symptoms rarely are. Leaning in to hear conversations and asking for repetitions are outward and rather obvious signs. My patients often confess to pretending to hear in social situations. They also dread getting caught out.

Skilled lipreaders can often conceal their hearing loss by putting the visual pieces of the puzzle together. However, hearing from another room or at other times when you can't see the speaker's face is likely to be an ongoing challenge. TV at a normal volume is difficult for most people with hearing loss, since quite often, you can't see the speaker's face. The magnitude of the required TV volume is often the tipping point that propels people to seek help. Spare a thought, too, for outward signs of cognitive load & weariness — hearing loss is tiring. Know that there are always discreet options, and the sooner you act, the better the outcome.

Elephant #4: "Don't hearing aids just end up in the top drawer?"

Unfortunately, there is some truth to that. In Australia, studies have shown that around a third of hearing aids almost never leave their case. Personally, I'm a stickler about reinforcing the need for full-time use, so over 90 percent of my patients wear their devices at least 12 hours per day. This is necessary to receive the full benefit from the hearing aids.

Elephant #5: "Don't hearing aids just make everything louder?"

Essentially, this is true for older, traditional beige banana devices and untrue for premium technology devices. Like much in modern life, we've all moved on.

Elephant #6: "I don't want to be sold something."

No one likes that feeling of being pressured into purchasing something, and that is not what you should expect when you attend a quality, independent audiology practice. Such practices, though few and far between, have a strong focus on patient education and depend very much on the word-of-mouth referrals from the patient base, which only comes as a result of effectively meeting patients' needs.

Most hearing practices these days are owned by foreign hearing aid manufacturers and retailers that typically have limited solutions to offer. Generally, you'll be able to determine whether a practice is independent because they will state it clearly on their website. Otherwise, just call and ask.

When investigating the right hearing specialist for you, make sure they have a focus on patient education rather than a pure focus on hearing aid devices. If you feel pressured to buy a device, I'd encourage you to politely move on and get a second opinion.

Regarding the cost, there are a range of options, none of which equate to more than $250 per month over a 3-year period, depending on the type of solution and technology level. The core considerations are ensuring that the solution is appropriate and beneficial enough to be worn for at least 12 hours per day and that you have confidence in the clinician making the recommendation.

Elephant #7: "I/my friend/a family member didn't have a great experience at another practice. Where to from here?"

Perhaps the staff at the other practice lacked confidence and experience, or were simply not at liberty to use their clinical judgement by virtue of their employment situation. The hearing industry in Australia is arguably the most corporatized in the world, meaning that most clinicians are frequently required to answer to a non-clinical boss. This trend appears to be increasing worldwide. These companies are often owned by hearing aid manufacturers, which means they're 'obliged' to offer only their products. In my experience, no single manufacturer has the ideal solution for all patients. Independent audiology practices are in the unique position of having access to the full range of solutions so they can recommend what's best for you.

Elephant #8: "Is this going to be a long, drawn-out process?"

Not at all. Most people with hearing loss walk out of their first appointment being able to hear better straight away. Remember that adjusting to your new world of sound is an adaptive process. Your audiologist should let you know what to expect and make the experience as comfortable for you as they can.

Today's premium devices require only the simple act of putting them in first thing in the morning and taking them off at night, with nothing to do in between but enjoy the benefits. Most devices are rechargeable, eliminating the hassle of having to change batteries, and they automatically adapt to changing acoustic environments without you lifting a finger.

A common inconvenience for hearing impaired people is mishearing in social settings to the point where they avoid them. Our job is to help avert that situation and enable a fuller participation in life.

Are you having problems hearing?
If so, those around you already know it.
Hearing loss is no laughing matter,
so don't be a punchline.

~Leslie Nielsen

CHAPTER 10

Tinnitus, the ring of discontent

Tinnitus, commonly known as 'ringing in the ears' affects approximately 10-15 percent of people on a regular basis, and around 18 percent of Australians and Americans are affected by it.

Most people think they're alone in experiencing it because it's not something that's typically discussed. No one goes out for coffee and says to their friends, "Hey, do you hear that high-pitched squeal?"

For some, tinnitus comes and goes without rhyme or reason, while for others, it's a constant companion. It tends to be more noticeable in a quiet environment, like when you're in bed at night trying to sleep. Another more disturbing, yet common, belief is that tinnitus is all in the mind, which is another reason people tend not to bring it up in general conversation. The truth is, tinnitus is absolutely not imagined.

What is tinnitus?

Tinnitus is most commonly experienced as a high-pitched ringing sound, but it can also be a whistling, hissing, blowing, buzzing, humming, sizzling, or roaring sound. The noises can be barely detectable, or they can be debilitatingly loud. The sounds of tinnitus don't exist in the external environment; only the sufferer can hear them, which is why it seems to be an imaginary condition.

You may have heard of phantom pain, which is when a person who has lost a limb reports that they can feel pain as if that limb was still there. Neuroscientists believe that since the brain is used to receiving sensory signals from that part of the body, when the signals cease, the brain steps in and generates its own 'phantom' signals around what the limb is experiencing. In the case of tinnitus that's caused by hearing loss, however mild or significant the loss, there's a similar mechanism at play. The brain is used to receiving auditory signals from the ear, and when they are no longer detected, or are greatly reduced, the brain generates its own signals or sounds to compensate. This is an undesirable dysfunction.

Who develops tinnitus?

Tinnitus can affect people of all ages, genders, races, and hearing abilities. Following are the most common risk factors:

Ageing: The older you get, the more the nerve fibers in your ears deteriorate, leading to gradual hearing loss and quite often, tinnitus.

Smoking: You have a higher risk of experiencing tinnitus if you smoke.

Gender: Though both men and women get tinnitus, the number of men who suffer the affliction is higher.

Cardiovascular issues: Those with high blood pressure or atherosclerosis (narrowed arteries) have an increased risk of tinnitus.

Exposure to loud noises: People who work in noisy places such as factories and airport tarmacs are more susceptible. Those exposed to loud music, such as at concerts or through excessively loud headphones, are more likely to suffer tinnitus.

What makes tinnitus worse?

For some people, tinnitus is only a mild annoyance, but sometimes, it may get worse.

There are three main factors that can exacerbate tinnitus:

Silence: The quieter the environment, the louder the tinnitus. Unfortunately, as mentioned previously, your brain is going to try to compensate for missing sounds, and in a quiet room, such as your bedroom at night, you may notice your tinnitus even more.

Sleep deprivation: Scientists across the world have documented that a lack of sleep worsens tinnitus.

Stress: To date, the exact link between tinnitus and stress isn't known, but they are undoubtedly related. When we're under stress, our bodies can experience a fight or flight response. This puts the body on high alert, and one of the ways it responds is by heightening our sense of hearing. Of course, that makes even low-level tinnitus more noticeable. Most sufferers report that their tinnitus is worse when they are stressed, and for many, their first experience of tinnitus was during a period of great stress.

What to do about tinnitus

It's important to note that there is no one-size-fits-all approach to tinnitus management, and recent research recommends a personalized approach under the guidance of an audiologist.

Following are some broad strategies that will help you:

One: Have your hearing checked. One of the most common causes of tinnitus is hearing loss. Even mild hearing loss can cause tinnitus, and many people are unaware their hearing has deteriorated because it usually happens so gradually. Make an appointment with an independent audiologist who will test your hearing with state-of-the-art medical equipment that will accurately diagnose your hearing.

Aside from providing you with a proper diagnosis, the audiologist will assist you with strategies to treat your tinnitus and reassure you about your specific situation. A word of warning though, consulting 'Dr. Google' may unearth some misleading claims about tinnitus that could cause you unnecessary concern.

Two: Avoid silence. It makes your tinnitus more noticeable. Some sufferers find that having the radio or TV on at a low volume can be helpful. White noise apps and devices designed to put babies to sleep can also help. The volume of the tinnitus sound will be reduced, relative to the background noise that you introduce. If using apps, the radio, or TV when going to sleep, check to see if your smartphone or other device has a sleep function that turns the sound off after a certain duration. Or, you may prefer to leave it on all night.

Three: Manage your stress. Find ways to reduce your stress, or if you can't avoid stressful situations, then work on ways to take the pressure off. Be kind to yourself, go for a walk, have a massage, listen to relaxing music, read a book or watch a comedy.

Is there a cure for tinnitus?

Unfortunately, there's no complete cure but treatments are effective. The goal is to take it from being troublesome and intrusive to something you may experience occasionally and less intensely.

If you or someone you care about are bothered by tinnitus, contact us for further information or visit our website at **www.neuaudio.com.au** where you can access additional tinnitus resources.

CHAPTER 11

Giving back – my pledge to change 1,000 lives in Cambodia

In Australia, there's a safety net for the less fortunate, with government programs to help children, indigenous populations, and older Australians on low incomes. The people of Cambodia are not so lucky. Cambodia is one of the poorest countries in the world. Around two million Cambodians live with disabling hearing loss, and it's estimated that 85 percent of those live in abject poverty.

Fewer than one percent of Cambodians who need hearing aids have them, primarily due to the cost. Only five percent of older Cambodians are eligible for any sort of pension, which means many have no choice but to continue working. Poor health (including hearing problems) directly affects their livelihoods, their capacity to care for children, and their ability to participate in daily life.

All Ears Cambodia is a small, non-government audiology charity based in Phnom Penh. What makes this organization unique is their focus on training local clinicians. Unlike other charities that fly in and out of third world countries as a once-off, the training and employment of local clinicians enables the continuity of care that makes a real difference over the long-term.

I've supported All Ears Cambodia since 2012. I've coordinated hearing device donations totaling over $75,000, sent pre-loved devices from my practices, and presented sessions as a guest lecturer for their audiology students at times when international travel is possible. During my visits, I tutor clinical staff on hearing device fittings. All proceeds from this book will be allocated to funding future teaching visits.

To learn more about All Ears Cambodia, please visit: **www.allearscambodia.org**

CHAPTER 12

My journey into audiology

I often tell a story at my Hearing and Brain Health seminars about an uncompromising performance coach who pressed me on the 'why' of what I do. She pushed me to be really clear about it. This helped me to set my priorities straight and maintain a sharp focus for my professional practice. My initial response to the 'why' question led me to recount the time I first became aware of audiology as a profession. I was studying undergraduate psychology at the time, and while learning about how all the senses work, I became fascinated with the ingenious and intricate sense of hearing. At the time, I was playing bass guitar in bands, and my background in music was no doubt partially responsible for this fascination.

My psychology lecturer taught us about the growing profession of audiology, and with emerging technologies, an ageing population, and a shortage of clinicians, the career prospects looked appealing. By this time, I had already concluded that counselling psychology wasn't for me. Back then it seemed to me that a counselling psychologist may never really know how much they've helped someone. By contrast, audiologists have the potential to change lives dramatically and measurably, quite often as early as at the initial appointment.

However, this answer was not enough for my stubborn coach. She wanted me to delve even deeper into my 'why'. So, we traversed back to my childhood for more clues regarding the source of my passion. I recalled a time when I was nine years old, and my grandfather (we called him Fardy) was visiting from Victoria. We were clearing out the bottom of the block surrounding our new family home at Samford, a semi-rural community north-west of Brisbane. I was the third of six children, and Fardy had tasked us all with transporting around 20 large logs and twice as many tires 100 meters up an extremely steep hill. The previous residents had horses and had used the logs for equestrian practice.

It was a hot and humid Queensland day. It took all six of us to haul the first log up the hill. Already suffering from splinters and aching legs after the first run, I figured there had to be a better way. I worked out that if I laid the log horizontally between two tires and rolled them up the hill it would be much easier. In fact, two young children could do this on their own. As a result, several hours of hard labor was reduced to a cruisy half hour.

Fardy pulled me aside and congratulated me on my solution. He told me if I studied hard, there would be no limits to what I could achieve. Do you think I listened to him? Well, not entirely. Growing up, I was a distracted student and likely a source of worry for my parents.

My grandfather was a stoic, charismatic man. He was a fourth-generation farm owner, the patriarch of the extended family including 24 grandchildren, and a pillar of his local community. He suffered from debilitating noise-induced hearing loss and tinnitus. His old-fashioned beige banana hearing aids were so uncomfortable and noisy that they never left his bedroom.

Unfortunately, Fardy's health deteriorated a short time after visiting us. He developed a range of conditions, including a stroke and the associated cognitive decline, before he passed away at age 81.

So how does this story relate to my 'why'? The reason I get up in the morning and do what I do is because I love problem solving—be it heavy logs, navigating a challenging hearing evaluation, or thinking of better ways to serve my patients. I get a thrill out of developing simple solutions to complex problems, communicating with people, and finding shortcuts that yield quality outcomes. This is not about being lazy or providing a substandard solution. It's about a logical, give me a lever and a place to stand and I will move the Earth, kind of motivation for me.

What I saw in audiology was a potential platform to deliver the ultimate shortcut to improving overall health. Once I discovered audiology, I needed to ensure that I was accepted into the Master of Audiology course, so I applied myself to my studies and achieved the highest grades for my remaining psychology subjects. My Master's thesis was titled, 'Quality of Life Improvement and Hearing Aids for Adults', which framed the focus of my future in the field. I finished in the top five percent of my class nearly 20 years ago and have specialized in and dedicated myself to hearing aids for adults ever since.

My first professional role was in a Brisbane practice working with a group of Ear, Nose and Throat specialists. This was a baptism of fire with respect to learning first-hand the lengths my patients would go to just to avoid wearing hearing aids. I understood that people generally hated the thought of them. For many, it was a sign of getting old and/or somehow being incapacitated. For others, hearing aids were uncomfortable and noisy, and at that time, they were primitive by today's standards. I found myself almost apologizing for what I was fitting.

The success of the devices was reasonable for quiet situations, but far from satisfactory in environments with background noise, which was usually where the patients needed the most help. What made matters worse was the fact that we worked with the ugly traditional beige bananas, which I refuse to work with these days. During my first year, I managed to negotiate my way to the corner office and doubled my salary, but I still wasn't fulfilled. I wasn't solving the problem of people's resistance to hearing device treatment, which was a source of daily frustration for me.

Then I managed to secure a position with a rapidly expanding, innovative company in New Zealand. I commenced a clinical role, and within a year, they had me working on the expansion of the company and innovative practice modalities. At that time, government funding for hearing aids was very generous for people with noise-induced hearing loss, which is quite common in New Zealand, with agriculture as the major industry. Plus, new technology had become available, and I was finally able to achieve more acceptable outcomes for my patients. I mainly fit open-fit hearing aids, which have a small body that sits above the ear and a light wire that leads into the ear canal. The old-style hearing aids had to be custom made by taking a molded impression of the ear. Their mechanisms were unrefined, and they were clunky to wear. Now, for the first time, the new technology enabled my patients to go home hearing better immediately.

The company was growing rapidly, and the owners asked me to start preparing to lead their expansion into Australia. As mentioned earlier, in Australia, people tend to avoid addressing hearing problems for seven to ten years on average. I realized that the fewer barriers you erect, the more likely people are to act.

Location was one such barrier. Audiology practices were traditionally relegated to small shopping strips or at the back end of hospitals, so I decided

Hearing & Brain Health

to investigate the possibility of convenient, high-foot-traffic shopping mall practices. This was a major benefit for the patients because they could combine their visits with other errands.

Our first shopping mall practice was in Tweed Heads on the Gold Coast. We had a high number of initial enquiries but relatively few appointments. To give patients a reason to book in, a talented Texan colleague and I developed touchscreen hearing screening technology that enabled us and the potential patient to determine hearing aid candidacy in around five minutes. This caused the practices to take off. Over the five years I was running the company, we grew to 35 practices. At the time of writing this, that company has over 100 practices and are screening approximately 160,000 Australians for hearing loss each year.

Following my time in Australia, I managed a multinational hearing care company in Singapore and Malaysia. Approximately 33 percent of people in Australia with hearing loss have hearing aids. In Singapore and Malaysia, that number is an alarming two percent. I discovered an unfortunate urban myth in Asia, where it's believed that the time to address a hearing loss is when you can't hear at all.

As a result, it was not uncommon to see people with 70-80 percent hearing loss attending our clinics for the first time. This magnitude of loss is exceptionally difficult to treat. Further, around half of my patients suffered from various degrees of cognitive decline. After five years in Asia, I was ready for a new challenge and secured a practice development role in the dynamic city of Nashville, Tennessee. My role was to support 250 independent private practices across Tennessee and Kentucky.

I enjoyed working with independent practice owners and observing the different ways in which they practiced audiology. The most successful and fulfilled practice owners had a strong focus on patient education, premium technology, and ongoing quality care. Their patients raved about them. It didn't take too long for me to start thinking about developing my own practices based on similar principles.

As an Australian, there are several barriers associated with starting a practice from scratch in the United States. In fact, it is more straightforward to start a practice in Australia and then expand to the United States. I saw that as a potential long-term goal, and after an exciting year in Nashville, I returned to my hometown of Brisbane to start my own practice there and later in Melbourne and the Gold Coast.

Relatively few independent practices exist in Australia. Nearly 90 percent are chains owned by multinational corporations with limitations on the technology they can offer. Please note that it is not my intention to denigrate other hearing health care professionals, I know first-hand that their treatment options and time restraints are often not their own choosing. It is my intention to give you the 'call a spade a spade' type of advice you'd expect from any trusted advisor.

*It is not the voice
that commands the story:
it is the ear.*

~Italo Calvino

CHAPTER 13

About my practice

My practice, NeuAudio – Hearing and Brain Health, focuses squarely on the principles outlined in this book. My ideal patient is someone who understands the consequences of untreated hearing loss, is proactive, and wants to live a life without limitation. Our profession has one of the lowest effective treatment rates for a major medical condition that I can find, which is why I do things differently.

One third of hearing aid users don't wear their devices at all or wear them for less than two hours a day, one third wear them only 2-12 hours per day, and one third wear them 12-plus hours a day, as they should. Given that only around 33 percent of Australians who need hearing aids have them, this equates to an effective treatment rate of approximately 17 percent. That same depressing figure applies to the United States as well. I challenge you to find a healthcare profession with a lower treatment rate. To emphasize further, merely getting a hearing test and/or owning hearing aids does not equate to effective treatment.

Any of my patients will tell you that I'm fanatical about full-time use of hearing technology. I want all my patients to achieve maximum value from their investment and to get the most out of life. Therefore, I only work with the best technology. I'm proud to say that over 90 percent of my patients wear their technology for more than 12 hours per day.

Consider the next cocktail party or family gathering you attend. Would you prefer to labor through conversations like hauling a heavy log with splinters up a steep hill in the heat, or roll on in and effortlessly engage with your loved ones? If the latter sounds like you, I guarantee your life will be better following your first appointment.

If you're interested in ongoing updates and advice, please visit www.neuaudio.com.au and/or join our Facebook community by liking our NeuAudio page.

I provide free Hearing and Brain health seminars at least once a month, both virtually and in person. If you know of anyone who may find the content interesting, please ask them to contact us for details about the next session.

If you missed the link to my totally free, online Hearing & Brain Health Academy mentioned earlier in this book, here it is again:

https://neuaudio.link/brainhealth

Presenting to community groups and retirement communities is one of my favorite activities, as such groups are frequently highly engaged and proactive. If you would like me to present at your organization or community group, please email **info@neuaudio.com.au** and we'll aim to make arrangements.

Academic References

Abrahamson J. Group audiologic rehabilitation. Seminars in Hearing. 2000;21:227–233.

Abrams, H., T. H. Chisolm, and R. McArdle. 2002. "A Cost-Utility Analysis of Adult Group Audiologic Rehabilitation: Are the Benefits Worth the Costs?" Journal of Rehabilitation Research and Development 39: 549–558.

Aldy, J. E., and W. K. Viscusi. 2008. "Adjusting the Value of a Statistical Life for Age and Cohort Effects." Review of Economics and Statistics 90: 573–581.

Andersson G, Melin L, Scott B, Lindberg P. An evaluation of a behavioral treatment approach to hearing impairment. Behavior Research Therapy. 1995;33:283–292.

Armstrong NM, An Y, Doshi J, et al. Association of midlife hearing impairment with late-life temporal lobe volume loss. JAMA Otolaryngol Head Neck Surg 2019; 145: 794.

Amieva H, Ouvrard C, Giulioli C, Meillon C, Rullier L, Dartigues JF. Self-reported hearing loss, hearing aids, and cognitive decline in elderly adults: a 25-Year Study. J Am Geriatr Soc 2015; 63: 2099–104.

Amieva H, Ouvrard C, Meillon C, Rullier L, Dartigues JF. Death, depression, disability, and dementia associated with self-reported hearing problems: a 25-year study. J Gerontol A Biol Sci Med Sci 2018; 73: 1383–89.

Astolfi P, Caselli G, Fioranic O, et al. Late reproduction behavior in Sardinia: spatial analysis suggests local aptitude towards reproductive longevity. Evolution and Human Behavior. 2009;30(2):93–102.

Barker F, Mackenzie E, Elliott L, Jones S, de Lusignan S. Interventions to improve hearing aid use in adult auditory rehabilitation. Cochrane Database Syst Rev. 2014 Jul 12;(7).

Beck DL. Inside the research: Auditory deprivation, brain changes secondary to hearing loss, and more: An interview with Anu Sharma, PhD. Hearing Review. 2017;24(1):40.

Bell L, Wagels L, Neuschaefer-Rube C, Fels J, Gur RE, Konrad K. The Cross-Modal Effects of Sensory Deprivation on Spatial and Temporal Processes in Vision and Audition: A Systematic Review on Behavioral and Neuroimaging Research since 2000. Neural Plast. 2019;2019:9603469.

Bernabei R, Bonuccelli U, Maggi S, et al, and the participants in the Workshop on Hearing Loss and Cognitive Decline in Older Adults. Hearing loss and cognitive decline in older adults: questions and answers. Aging Clin Exp Res 2014; 26: 567–73.

Blustein, J., and B. E. Weinstein. 2016b. "Blustein and Weinstein Respond" to the Letter by Stein, Z.A.,"The Hearing Aid Industry Is More Helpful than Suggested." American Journal of Public Health 106: e1.

Cabral J, Tonocchi R, Ribas Â, Almeida G, Rosa M, Massi G, Berberian AP. The efficacy of hearing aids for emotional and auditory tinnitus issues. Int Tinnitus J. 2016 Jul 22;20(1):54-8.

Carniel CZ, Sousa JCF, Silva CDD, Fortunato-Queiroz CAU,

Hyppolito MÂ, Santos PLD. Implications of using the Hearing Aids on quality of life of elderly Codas. 2017 Oct 19;29(5)

Caselli G, Lipsi RM. Survival differences among the oldest old in Sardinia: who, what, where, and why. Demographic Research. 2006;14:267–294.

Chen Z, Yuan W. Central plasticity and dysfunction elicited by aural deprivation in the critical period. Front Neural Circuits. 2015;9:26. Published 2015 Jun 2.

Cheung SW, Bonham BH, Schreiner CE, Godey B, Copenhaver DA. Realignment of interaural cortical maps in asymmetric hearing loss. J Neurosci 2009; 29: 7065–78.

Cunningham DR. Hearing aid selection counseling: helping patients make decisions. The Hearing Journal. 1996;49:31–49.

Darrow, K. Stop Living In Isolation: How Treating Hearing Loss & Tinnitus can change your life, maintain your independence, and may reduce your risk of dementia. 2017.

Davis A, Smith P, Ferguson M, Stephens D, Gianopoulos I. Acceptability, benefit and costs of early screening for hearing disability: a study of potential screening tests and models. Health Technol Assess 2007; 11: 1–294.

De Silva, D. G., N. Thakurb, and M. Xiec. 2013. "A Hedonic Price Analysis of Hearing Aid Technology." Applied Economics 45: 2315–2323.

Deal JA, Betz J, Yaffe K, et al, for the Health ABC Study Group. Hearing impairment and incident dementia and cognitive decline in older adults: the Health ABC Study. J

Gerontol A Biol Sci Med Sci 2016; published online April 12.

Deal JA, Sharrett AR, Albert MS, et al. Hearing impairment and cognitive decline: a pilot study conducted within the atherosclerosis risk in communities neurocognitive study. Am J Epidemiol 2015; 181: 680–90.

Donohue, A., J. R. Dubno, and L. Beck. 2010. "Accessible and Affordable Hearing Health Care for Adults with Mild to Moderate Hearing Loss." Ear and Hearing 31: 2–6.

Fortunato, S., F. Forli, V. Guglielmi, G. Paludetti, S. Berrentini, and A.R. Fetoni. 2016. "A Review of New Insights on the Association between Hearing Loss and Cognitive Decline in Ageing." Acta Otorhinolaryngolica Italica 36:155–166.

Fritze T, Teipel S, Óvári A, Kilimann I, Witt G, Doblhammer G. Hearing impairment affects dementia incidence. An analysis based on longitudinal health claims data in Germany. PLoS One 2016; 11: e0156876.

Garnefski N, Kraaij V. Cognitive coping and goal adjustment are associated with symptoms of depression and anxiety in people with acquired hearing loss. International Journal of Audiology. 2012;51:545–550.

Garraghty PE, Kaas JH. Neuroplasticity of the adult primate auditory cortex following cochlear hearing loss Am J Otol 1993; 14: 252–58.

Gatehouse S. Rehabilitation: identification of needs, priorities and expectations, and the evaluation of benefit. International Journal of Audiology. 2003;42:77–83.

Gates GA, Beiser A, Rees TS, D'Agostino RB, Wolf PA. Central auditory dysfunction may precede the onset of clinical dementia in people with probable Alzheimer's disease. J Am Geriatr Soc 2002; 50: 482–88.

Gates GA. Central presbycusis: an emerging view. Otolaryngol Head Neck Surg 2012; 147: 1–2.

Gates GA, Cobb JL, Linn RT, Rees T, Wolf PA, D'Agostino RB. Central auditory dysfunction, cognitive dysfunction, and dementia in older people. Arch Otolaryngol Head Neck Surg 1996; 122: 161–67.

Glick HA, Sharma A. Cortical neuroplasticity and cognitive function in early-stage, mild-moderate hearing loss: Evidence of neurocognitive benefit from hearing aid use. Front Neurosci. 2020;14:93.

Golub JS, Brickman AM, Ciarleglio AJ, Schupf N, Luchsinger JA. Association of subclinical hearing loss with cognitive performance. JAMA Otolaryngol Head Neck Surg 2019; 146: 57–67.

Gopinath B, Wang JJ, Schneider J, et al. Depressive symptoms in older adults with hearing impairments: the Blue Mountains Study. J Am Geriatr Soc 2009; 57: 1306–08.

Gurgel RK, Ward PD, Schwartz S, Norton MC, Foster NL, Tschanz JT. Relationship of hearing loss and dementia: a prospective, population-based study. Otol Neurotol 2014; 35: 775–81.

Gussekloo J, de Bont LE, von Faber M, et al. Auditory rehabilitation of older people from the general population – the Leiden 85-plus study. The British Journal of General Practice: The Journal of the Royal College of General

Practitioners. 2003;53:536–540.

Hallberg LRM, Hallberg U, Kramer SE. Self-reported hearing difficulties, communication strategies and psychological general well-being (quality of life) in patients with acquired hearing impairment. Disability and Rehabilitation. 2008;30:203–212.

Hartley D, Rochtchina E, Newall P, Golding M, Mitchell P. Use of hearing AIDS and assistive listening devices in an older Australian population. J Am Acad Audiol 2010; 21: 642–53.

Hengen J, Hammarström IL, Stenfelt S. Perceived Voice Quality and Voice-Related Problems Among Older Adults With Hearing Impairments J Speech Lang Hear Res. 2018 Sep 19;61(9).

Hong T, Mitchell P, Burlutsky G, Liew G, Wang JJ. Visual Impairment, Hearing Loss and Cognitive Function in an Older Population: Longitudinal Findings from the Blue Mountains Eye Study. PLoS One 2016; 11: e0147646.

Huang CQ, Dong BR, Lu ZC, Yue JR, Liu QX. Chronic diseases and risk for depression in old age: a meta-analysis of published literature. Ageing Res Rev 2010; 9: 131–41.

Kaplan-Neeman R, Muchnik C, Hildesheimer M, Henkin Y. Hearing aid satisfaction and use in the advanced digital era. Laryngoscope. 2012 Sep;122(9):2029-36.

Kakigi A, Hirakawa H, Harel N, Mount RJ, Harrison RV. Tonotopic mapping in auditory cortex of the adult chinchilla with amikacin-induced cochlear lesions. Audiology 2000; 39: 153–60.

Schwaber MK, Kelly-Campbell RJ, Lessoway K. Hearing aid and hearing assistance technology use in Aotearoa/New Zealand. Int J Audiol. 2015 May;54(5):308-15.

Kiely KM, Gopinath B, Mitchell P, Luszcz M, Anstey KJ. Cognitive, health, and sociodemographic predictors of longitudinal decline in hearing acuity among older adults. J Gerontol A Biol Sci Med Sci 2012; 67: 997–1003.

Kochkin, S. MarkeTrak VII: Hearing Loss Population Tops 31 Million People, The Hearing Review, Vol. 12(7) July 2005, pp. 16-29. Download: http://www.betterhearing.org/pdfs/MarkeTrak7_Koch kin_July05.pdf

Kochkin, S. & Rogin, C. Quantifying the Obvious: The Impact of Hearing Aids on Quality of Life, The Hearing Review, Vol 7(1) January 2000, pp. 8-34. Download: http://www.betterhearing.org/pdfs/ MR40.pdf

Lin FR, Metter EJ, O'Brien RJ, Resnick SM, Zonderman AB, Ferrucci L. Hearing loss and incident dementia. Arch Neurol 2011; 68: 214–20.

Gallacher J, Ilubaera V, Ben-Shlomo Y, et al. Auditory threshold, phonologic demand, and incident dementia. Neurology 2012; 79: 1583–90.

Lin FR, Ferrucci L, Metter EJ, An Y, Zonderman AB, Resnick SM. Hearing loss and cognition in the Baltimore Longitudinal Study of Aging. Neuropsychology 2011; 25: 763–70.

Lin FR. Hearing loss and cognition among older adults in the United States. J Gerontol A Biol Sci Med Sci 2011; 66: 1131–36.

Lin MY, Gutierrez PR, Stone KL, et al, and the Study of Osteoporotic Fractures Research Group. Vision impairment and combined vision and hearing impairment predict cognitive and functional decline in older women. J Am Geriatr Soc 2004; 52: 1996–2002.

Lin FR, Albert M. Hearing loss and dementia—who is listening? Aging Ment Health 2014; 18: 671–73. Livingston G, Sommerlad A, Orgeta V, et al. Dementia prevention, intervention, and care. Lancet. 2017;390(10113).

Livingston G, Huntley J, Sommerlad A, et al. Dementia prevention, intervention, and care: 2020 report of the Lancet Commission. Lancet. 2020 Aug 8;396.

Long P, Wan G, Roberts MT, Corfas G. Myelin development, plasticity, and pathology in the auditory system. Dev Neurobiol. 2018;78(2).

Loughrey DG, Kelly ME, Kelley GA, Brennan S, Lawlor BA. Association of age-related hearing loss with cognitive function, cognitive impairment, and dementia: a systematic review and meta-analysis. JAMA Otolaryngol Head Neck Surg 2018; 144: 115–26.

Maharani A, Dawes P, Nazroo J, Tampubolon G, Pendleton N. Longitudinal relationship between hearing aid use and cognitive function in older Americans. J Am Geriatr Soc 2018; 66: 1130–36.

McCoy SL, Tun PA, Cox LC, Colangelo M, Stewart RA, Wingfield A. Hearing loss and perceptual effort: downstream effects on older adults' memory for speech. Q J Exp Psychol A 2005; 58: 22–33.

Mondelli MF, Souza PJ. Quality of life in elderly adults before and after hearing aid fitting. Braz J Otorhinolaryngol. 2012 Jun;78(3):49-56.

Nieman CL, Marrone N, Mamo SK, et al. The Baltimore HEARS Pilot Study: an affordable, accessible, community-delivered hearing care intervention. Gerontologist 2016; published online Dec 7.

Pereira-Jorge M.R, et al. Anatomical and Functional MRI Changes after One Year of Auditory Rehabilitation with Hearing Aids. Neural Plasticity. 2018 Sep; 9303674.

Pienaar E, Stearn N, Swanepoel de W. Self-reported outcomes of aural rehabilitation for adult hearing aid users in a South African context. S Afr J Commun Disord. 2010 Dec;57:4, 6, 8.

Poulain M, Pes G, Salaris L. A population where men live as long as women: villagrande strisaili, sardinia. J Aging Res. 2011;2011:153756.

Ray J, Popli G, Fell G. Association of cognition and age-related hearing impairment in the English longitudinal study of ageing. JAMA Otolaryngol Head Neck Surg 2018; 144: 876–82.

Rezende BA, Lemos SMA, Medeiros AM. Quality of life of children with poor school performance: association with hearing abilities and behavioral issues Arq Neuropsiquiatr. 2019 Mar;77(3):147-154.

Ribeiro UASL, Souza VC, Lemos SMA Quality of life and social determinants in individual hearing AIDS users Codas. 2019 Apr 1;31(2).

Rockhill B, Newman B, Weinberg C. Use and misuse of population attributable fractions. Am J Public Health 1998; 88: 15–19.

Health and Social Care Information Centre. Health Survey for England 2014: health, social care and lifestyles: summary of key findings. London: Health and Social Care Information Centre, 2015.

Scholes S, Mindell J. Health Survey for England 2014: health, social care and lifestyles. In: Craig R, Fuller E, Mindell J, eds. Chapter 4: Hearing. London: Health and Social Care Information Centre, 2014.

Sharma A, Glick H. Cortical neuroplasticity in hearing loss: Why it matters in clinical decision-making for children and adults. Hearing Review. 2018;25(7):20-24.

Sinha UK, Hollen KM, Rodriguez R, Miller CA. Auditory system degeneration in Alzheimer's disease. Neurology 1993; 43: 779–85.

Subramanian SV, Kim D, Kawachi I. Covariation in the socioeconomic determinants of self-rated health and happiness: a multivariate multilevel analysis of individuals and communities in the USA. J Epidemiol Community Health. 2005;59(8):664-669.

Valentijn SAM, van Boxtel MPJ, van Hooren SAH, et al. Change in sensory functioning predicts change in cognitive functioning: results from a 6-year follow-up in the maastricht aging study. J Am Geriatr Soc 2005; 53: 374–80.

Vanderauwera J, Hellemans E, Verhaert N. Research Insights on Neural Effects of Auditory Deprivation and Restoration in Unilateral Hearing Loss: A Systematic Review. J Clin Med. 2020;9(3):812. Published 2020 Mar 17.

Waldinger RJ, Schulz MS. What's love got to do with it? Social functioning, perceived health, and daily happiness in married octogenarians. Psychol Aging. 2010;25(2):422-431.

WHO. 2017 "Global Costs of Unaddressed Hearing Loss and Cost-Effectiveness of Interventions." A WHO Report, 2017. Geneva: World Health Organization. License: CC BY-NC-SA 3.0 IGO.

Author Contact

Email   info@neuaudio.com.au

Website   www.neuaudio.com.au

Instagram   instagram.com/neuaudio

Facebook   facebook.com/neuaudio

Linkedin   linkedin.com/in/andrew-campbell-
            9b543923/

Acknowledgments

A big thanks to my talented team and to those who have inspired this book, including Samantha Brooks, Joanne Campbell, Michael Collas-Smith, Professor Louise Hickson, Peter Hutson, Anya Hutson, Jeanette Leigh, Brian James, Dr. Doug Maher, Jeffrey Pang and Nicole Turley.

CPSIA information can be obtained
at www.ICGtesting.com
Printed in the USA
BVHW021523080922
646511BV00002B/10